Eating Smart & Living Strong:

A Practical Guide

To

Lifelong Health

By

Richard A. Regan

Table of Contents

Introduction 5

Chapter 1 11

The Power of Nutrition 11

Chapter 2 28

Creating a Personalized Nutrition Plan
.... 28

Chapter 3 45

Meals Planning 45

Chapter 4 69

Mindful Eating 69

Chapter 5 84

Cooking for Health and Flavor 84

Chapter 6 95

Eating Smart on the Go 95

Chapter 7 103

Hydration and Wellness 103

Chapter 8 118

Fitness and Nutrition Synergy........ 118

Chapter 9 128

Special Dietary Consideration....... 128

Chapter 10 143

Consistency with Healthy Eating.... 143

Chapter 11 153

Taking Your Health to the Next Level
.... 153

Chapter 12 168

How to Stay Healthy for Life 168

Conclusion 174

Introduction

In the hustle and bustle of our fast-paced lives, it is all too easy to lose sight of the most essential element that fuels our journey, which is our health. Our bodies are remarkable vessels, requiring the right nourishment to thrive and endure the challenges that come our way. Yet, amidst the constant stream of information and fad diets, finding a solid path toward lifelong health can feel like a daunting task.

But fear not, for within these pages lies a transformative guide to lead you on a journey of self-discovery and empowerment welcome to "Eating Smart, Living Strong." This book is not just another fleeting dieting trend but a comprehensive and practical approach to nurturing your body and revitalizing your spirit.

Chapter by chapter, we will explore nutrition that goes beyond mere calorie counting and restrictive eating. Here, we delve into the heart of the matter, uncovering the power of nutrition and its profound impact on our overall well-being. From understanding the fundamental nutrients that sustain us to crafting personalized meal plans that align with your unique lifestyle, you will gain the knowledge to make informed choices that nurture your body, mind, and soul.

"Grocery shopping" will take on a new meaning as you learn to discern between nutritious choices and the hidden pitfalls of the supermarket aisles. With this newfound wisdom, you will create delectable meals that satiate your taste buds and nourish your body with the goodness it deserves.

Beyond the plate, we will explore the deeper connections between our minds and our eating habits in the chapter on "Mindful Eating." Discover the art of savoring each bite, the pleasure of being present at the moment, and the liberation from emotional eating that will elevate your dining experience to a whole new level.

Whether you are a culinary novice or a seasoned home cook, "Cooking for Health and Flavor" will inspire you to embrace the magic of the kitchen. From simple yet nutritious recipes to the art of balancing flavors with herbs and spices, you will become the master of your culinary destiny, all while nourishing your body with meals made from the heart.

But what about those moments when life takes us on the go? "Eating Smart on the Go" will equip you with the tools to make healthy choices when dining out, traveling, or simply snacking during your busy day. No longer will you feel at the mercy of unhealthy temptations; instead, you will hold the power to sustain your vitality wherever you may be.

Throughout this transformative journey, we will also explore the synergy between nutrition and fitness. You will learn how to optimize your performance by pairing your physical activity with the right fuel, propelling you toward your fitness goals with newfound vigor.

As we progress, we will address special dietary considerations, embracing the diversity of individual needs and exploring how to cater to various dietary preferences and restrictions. Whether you are a devoted vegetarian, face gluten sensitivities, or navigate the ever-changing dietary needs of different life stages, this book will provide insights and solutions to nourish your body in the most mindful and respectful manner.

Yet, true wellness extends beyond the physical realm. In "Overcoming Challenges and Staying Consistent," we will delve into the art of perseverance and celebrate the victories, no matter how small. From handling setbacks gracefully to inspiring others to embark on their health journey, you will become a beacon of strength and knowledge.

As you turn the pages of this book, remember that the path to lifelong health is not a rigid road but a dynamic and beautiful evolution. The knowledge you acquire will be the compass guiding you toward a life filled with strength, energy, and joy. Your health journey will be unique, your experiences your own, and the destination—more vibrant and invigorating than you ever imagined.

So, let us begin this transformative odyssey together—where "Eating Smart, Living Strong" is not merely a choice but a celebration of the remarkable gift of life that resides within you. Let us embrace the power of nutrition, enrich our lives, and nourish our souls as we embark on this journey of discovery, empowerment, and lasting well-being.

Chapter 1

The Power of Nutrition

Understanding the Role of Nutrition in Overall Health

Nutrition plays an important role in overall health and well-being. The food we consume provides our bodies with essential nutrients, which are needed for the growth, development, and maintenance of bodily functions. A balanced and nutritious diet is vital for maintaining a healthy body and preventing various health conditions. Here are some key aspects of how nutrition impacts overall health:

Energy and Metabolism: Food provides energy for daily activities and bodily functions. The body breaks down the nutrients in food into energy through metabolism. Carbohydrates, fats, and proteins are macronutrients that provide energy.

Growth and Development: Adequate nutrition is critical for proper growth and development, especially during childhood, adolescence, and pregnancy. Nutrients like proteins, vitamins, minerals, and essential fatty acids support the formation of tissues, bones, and organs.

Immune Function: A well-balanced diet with essential vitamins and minerals, such as vitamin C, vitamin D, zinc, and selenium, helps strengthen the immune system. A robust immune system can better defend the body against infections and illnesses.

Maintaining a Healthy Weight: Proper nutrition is essential for maintaining a healthy weight. A balanced diet that includes appropriate portion sizes and a variety of nutrient-rich foods helps prevent obesity and related health issues.

Heart Health: A diet low in saturated and trans fats, cholesterol, and sodium can help reduce the risk of heart disease. Foods rich in fiber, such as fruits, vegetables, and whole grains, can also support heart health.

Digestive Health: A diet high in fiber promotes good digestive health by preventing constipation and supporting a healthy gut microbiome. Probiotics, found in fermented foods like yogurt, also contribute to a balanced gut.

Bone Health: Adequate intake of calcium, vitamin D, and other minerals is essential for maintaining strong and healthy bones, reducing the risk of osteoporosis and fractures.

Cognitive Function: Certain nutrients, such as omega-3 fatty acids, antioxidants, and vitamins, may play a role in brain health and cognitive function. These nutrients are found in foods like fish, nuts, seeds, and fruits.

Mental Health: There is growing evidence to suggest that nutrition can influence mental health. Consuming a diet rich in whole foods and nutrients, such as omega-3 fatty acids and B vitamins, may positively impact mood and reduce the risk of depression and anxiety.

Disease Prevention: A balanced diet can help reduce the risk of chronic diseases such as type 2 diabetes, certain cancers, and hypertension.

To maintain overall health through nutrition, it's essential to follow a balanced diet that includes a variety of nutrient-dense foods. This means incorporating a wide range of fruits, vegetables, whole grains, lean proteins, healthy fats, and dairy or dairy alternatives. Additionally, limiting the intake of processed foods, sugary beverages, and foods high in saturated and trans fats is crucial for optimal health.

It's important to note that individual nutritional needs can vary based on factors such as age, gender, activity level, and health conditions. Consulting with a registered dietitian or healthcare professional can help develop personalized nutrition plans to meet specific health goals.

Essential Nutrients

Essential nutrients are the vital components found in the foods we eat that are necessary for the proper functioning and health of our bodies. Here's a brief overview of the five major categories of essential nutrients:

Carbohydrates: Carbohydrates are the body's primary source of energy. When consumed, they are metabolized into glucose, a form of sugar, which our cells utilize to generate energy. Sugars like glucose and fructose belong to the category of simple carbohydrates. Complex carbohydrates are present in foods like grains and legumes. Excellent sources of complex carbohydrates that provide essential fiber, vitamins, and minerals include whole grains, fruits, vegetables, and legumes. Maintaining a healthy diet requires the consumption of these nutrient-rich foods.

Proteins: The growth, repair, and maintenance of body tissues heavily rely on proteins. The building blocks of proteins are amino acids. The body cannot produce nine essential amino acids on its own. It must obtain them from the diet. Animal sources like meat, fish, eggs, and dairy products are complete proteins containing all essential amino acids. Beans, lentils, nuts, and seeds are examples of plant-based sources that can provide proteins. Combining different plant sources may become necessary to obtain all essential amino acids.

Fats: Supporting cell structure is a vital role played by dietary fats, which are a concentrated source of energy. They also help in absorbing fat-soluble vitamins (A, D, E, and K) and producing important hormones. Avocados, nuts, seeds, and olive oil are examples of foods that contain unsaturated fats, which are widely recognized as heart-healthy and beneficial. Moderation is advised when consuming saturated fats, which can be found in animal products and certain plant oils. In order to maintain good health, it is best to avoid consuming trans fats which are frequently present in processed and fried foods.

Vitamins: They are crucial for different bodily processes. vitamins are organic compounds. They are classified into two groups: Vitamin C and B-complex vitamins are both water-soluble vitamins. In the other group, you can find fat-soluble vitamins like vitamins A, D, E, and K. Vitamin E acts as an antioxidant.

Minerals: Minerals are essential inorganic elements that perform various physiological functions. Some essential minerals include calcium, iron, magnesium, potassium, and zinc. They support nerve function, aiding in enzymatic reactions, carry oxygen in the blood, and maintaining strong bones are all crucial.

Including a variety of nutrient-dense foods in your diet is crucial for obtaining adequate amounts of essential nutrients. Consequently, placing importance on a broad selection of foods in our everyday meals is essential. Obtaining essential nutrients for optimal health requires the consumption of a diverse array of foods from different food groups.

Meeting the specific nutritional requirements of certain groups, such as pregnant women, children, and the elderly, might necessitate specific attention. A registered dietitian or healthcare professional can assist in creating personalized nutrition plans tailored to individual needs and health goals. Seeking guidance from qualified experts is essential for customizing the nutrition plan to meet specific requirements and objectives.

Optimizing macronutrients intake for peak performance and overall well-being

Achieving optimal performance and wellness requires a balanced intake of macronutrients. is crucial for reaching your highest potential both physically and mentally. The essential macronutrients include carbohydrates, proteins, and fats, and each has a designated role in maintaining bodily functions. Here are some guidelines for balancing macros for improved performance and overall health:

Carbohydrates

The body relies on carbohydrates as its main fuel. For both physical activity and brain function, the required fuel is supplied by them. Ensure that you include complex carbs obtained from whole grains, fruits, vegetables, and legumes within the context of your eating habits. These sources provide additional fiber, vitamins, and minerals compared to simple carbohydrates.

Prioritize unprocessed or minimally processed carbohydrates to avoid excessive added sugars and refined flour. The necessary carbohydrates depend on how active you are and your personal objectives. Those who participate in rigorous exercise and people actively involved in demanding physical activities potentially need additional carbs to effectively support the energy requirements of their activities.

Proteins

Muscle repair, tissue maintenance, and immune support all heavily rely on the function of proteins. It is important to have multiple options for protein sources in your diet, like lean meats such as chicken and turkey along with fish and dairy products.

In case you are involved in physical activity or participating in strength training, consider consuming slightly more protein to support muscle recovery and growth. However, excessive protein intake may not always be advantageous ultimately leading to potential kidney strain.

Fats

The production of hormones depends on dietary fats, fat-soluble vitamin uptake, and providing long-lasting fuel.

Pay attention to nourishing unsaturated fats among which are avocados, nuts, seeds, olive oil, and fatty fish.

Reduce the intake of saturated fats found in animal-based products and specific processed food items. Make sure to eliminate trans fats entirely, since they can harm your health.

Even though fat is vital, it contains a high number of calories, hence, take care of the serving sizes, particularly if you have weight management as an objective.

Micronutrients

Don't overlook the essential vitamins and minerals that help with various bodily functions, alongside macronutrients.

Consume a diverse range of fruits and vegetables to ensure you're getting a wide spectrum of micronutrients.

Consider taking a multivitamin if you have specific dietary restrictions or limitations. In addition, reaching out to a healthcare provider can help tackle any potential deficiencies.

Hydration

Temperature regulation, digestion, and nutrient transport all depend on water.

Make sure to consume an ample amount of water all day long. Pay attention to your body's thirst signals, especially during physical activity. Being adequately hydrated is essential for overall health and maximizing performance

Individualization

Each person's nutritional needs are unique, depending on factors such as age, gender, weight, activity level, and specific health goals.

Consider consulting with a registered dietitian or nutritionist to create a personalized nutrition plan that aligns with your individual needs and objectives.

Balancing macros and focusing on whole, nutrient-dense foods will contribute to improved performance, enhanced energy levels, and better overall wellness. Remember that maintaining a balanced and sustainable diet is key to long-term success.

Chapter 2

Creating a Personalized Nutrition Plan

Meeting your specific needs, goals, and preferences is crucial when it comes to creating a personalized nutrition plan. Here are the steps to develop a customized nutrition plan:

Assess Your Current Diet and Lifestyle

Make sure to observe your current eating patterns. This encompasses the kinds of foods you typically consume and the regularity of your eating habits.

Analyze your activity level and exercise routine to determine your energy requirements.

Set Clear Goals

Define your specific targets for improving your health and wellness. No matter the objective - be it weight management, enhancing athletic performance, managing a health condition, or simply embracing a healthier lifestyle. Having clear objectives will guide your nutrition plan.

Calculate Your Nutritional Requirements

If you want to estimate your daily caloric needs, you can rely on resources such as online calculators or professional advice from a registered dietitian. Ensure to consider your age, gender, weight, height, activity level, and goals. In addition, it is crucial to consider any particular dietary limitations or health conditions that might affect your caloric needs.

Establish the suitable macronutrient proportion (carbohydrates, proteins, and fats) depending on your objectives and personal choices.

Identify Macronutrient Ratios

You can modify the macronutrient distribution in your diet based on your goals. To illustrate, athletes may necessitate a higher consumption of carbohydrates to power their training. While those focused on weight loss might emphasize protein intake to support satiety and muscle maintenance.

Choose Nutrient-Dense Foods

Select whole, nutrient-rich foods that offer necessary vitamins, minerals, and fiber. Incorporate a variety of colorful fruits, vegetables, whole grains, lean proteins, healthy fats, and dairy or dairy alternatives into your meals. This is to guarantee a balanced and nutritious diet.

Consider Meal Timing and Frequency

Arrange your meals and snacks to align with your daily timetable and energy necessities. Certain individuals opt for three substantial meals, whereas others find smaller, more frequent meals advantageous.

Pay attention to meal timing around exercise to ensure you have enough energy for physical activity. Ensure proper recovery support afterward as well.

Stay Hydrated

Incorporate appropriate hydration into your nutritional strategy. Ensure proper hydration by drinking water throughout the day, adapting the quantity to match your activity level and the prevailing climate.

Account for Dietary Restrictions and Preferences

Be mindful of any dietary restrictions or food allergies you may possess. Find alternative choices that meet your nutrient demands.

Account for your food preferences and discover ways to include enjoyable foods in your plan to maintain adherence.

Monitor and Adjust

Track your advancement towards your objectives and make changes to your nutrition strategy as required.

When in doubt about specific elements of your plan or facing difficulties, consult a registered dietitian for advice. Personalized advice and support can be offered by them.

A sustainable nutrition plan should be enjoyable, flexible, and aligned with your lifestyle. Avoid extreme diets or fads. Maintenance of these diets can be challenging over time and they may not offer all the essential nutrients for optimal well-being. Prioritize a balanced and personalized approach to nutrition for lasting results.

Analyzing your existing eating habits and lifestyle

Evaluating your current eating habits and lifestyle is vital in order to gain insight into how they may be influencing your overall health and well-being. Engaging in self-reflection enables you to identify any areas that may need improvement and make the necessary adjustments to support a more wholesome way of living. Here are some key aspects to consider when evaluating your eating habits and lifestyle:

Food Choices

Remember to observe the varieties of food you normally have. Are the main food sources for them primarily whole, nutrient-dense foods like fruits, vegetables, whole grains, lean proteins, and healthy fats? Are you opting for processed and unhealthy options more often?

Take care to monitor your consumption of sugary foods, refined carbohydrates, saturated and trans fats, and sodium. Health can be negatively impacted by consuming these excessively.

Include adequate water intake as a part of your nutrition plan. Drink water throughout the day and adjust based on your activity level and climate.

Eating Environment

Reflect on your eating environment. Are you frequently eating while engaged in other activities like watching TV or working on the computer? Promoting a calm environment and engaging in mindful eating can support the cultivation of healthier dietary habits.

Physical Activity

Rate your level of physical activity. What type and intensity of exercise are you regularly participating in?

Incorporate both structured exercise like gym workouts or playing sports, and incidental activity such as walking or opting for stairs, into your lifestyle.

Stress and Emotional Eating

Pay attention to any recurring emotional eating behaviors. In response to stress, boredom, and other emotions, do you find yourself eating?

Developing healthier coping strategies can be facilitated by identifying triggers for emotional eating.

Sleep Patterns

Assess your sleep quality and duration. Poor sleep can impact hunger hormones and affect food choices.

Social and Cultural Influences

Take into account how social gatherings, cultural practices, and family traditions may shape your eating patterns and food selections.

Existing Health Conditions

Factor in any current health conditions or dietary limitations that might influence the food options you make.

Nutrient Intake

Evaluate your intake of vital nutrients, like vitamins, minerals, and macronutrients (carbs, proteins, and fats).

Eating Out and Food Preparation

Reflect on how frequently you visit restaurants and the specific food choices you usually make when dining outside.

Reflect on your food preparation habits. Do you prepare meals at your residence, or do you depend more on pre-packaged and processed foods?

Mental and Emotional Well-being

Consider your overall psychological and emotional wellness, as these elements can affect your eating patterns.

Insight into areas that may require improvement or adjustment can be obtained by assessing these aspects of your eating habits and lifestyle. Recognizing and understanding oneself is vital for implementing positive transformations that contribute to better health and well-being. If you discover areas that you'd like to enhance, think about establishing attainable and realistic goals to slowly incorporate modifications in your diet and lifestyle. If you're looking for customized guidance, it would be beneficial to consult with a registered dietitian or healthcare professional who can offer expert advice and assistance tailored to your unique requirements and aspirations.

Setting Realistic Goals for a Sustainable Healthy Diet

Setting realistic goals is crucial for adopting a sustainable and healthy diet. Long-term maintenance is possible through plan creation. Here are some tips to help you establish achievable objectives:

Identify Your Priorities: Figure out the exact elements of your diet and health that you aim to enhance. Whether it's weight management, better energy levels, improved heart health, or overall well-being. Being aware of your priorities allows you to prioritize the goals that are most relevant and important.

Be Specific and Measurable: Set clear and measurable goals. Define what eating healthier means in your own terms instead of keeping it vague. An alternative goal could be to limit soda consumption to once a week.

Start Small: Rather than attempting drastic changes all at once, begin with small, manageable goals. Building new habits over time is more sustainable through gradual adjustments.

Use the SMART Method: Utilize the SMART technique for setting objectives: Specific, Measurable, Attainable, Relevant, and Time-bound. This method aids in making sure that your objectives are clearly defined and achievable in a reasonable time frame.

Focus on Whole Foods: Increase your intake of whole, nutrient-dense foods. Put an emphasis on fresh produce, whole grains, lean proteins, and healthy fats, and steer clear of processed foods.

Practice mindful eating by being aware of your hunger and fullness cues. To reduce overeating and increase satisfaction, keep your attention on your food and take your time enjoying each bite.

Plan and Prepare: To avoid making unhealthy decisions at the last minute, schedule your meals and snacks in advance. Prepare wholesome meals and snacks to have on hand for emergencies.

Limit processed foods and added sugars: Reduce your consumption of processed foods and added sugars gradually. Read food labels and be mindful of hidden sugars in packaged products.

Be Patient and Flexible: Understand that adopting a healthy diet is a journey with ups and downs. Be patient with yourself and be willing to adjust your goals as needed.

Keep in mind that lasting change takes time and that obstacles are a normal part of the journey. Celebrate each accomplishment and place more emphasis on progress than perfection. If you run into problems or feel like you need more direction, think about speaking with a registered dietitian or nutritionist who can offer you specialized guidance and support to help you reach your objectives.

Making smart food choices and reading labels is essential for maintaining a healthy diet and ensuring you're consuming nutritious foods. Here are some tips to help you make informed choices and understand food labels:

Chapter 3

Meals Planning

Smart Food Choices and Reading Labels

Choosing the right foods to eat and understanding the information on food labels is important. When we make smart food choices, we are selecting foods that are good for our bodies. This means choosing foods that are nutritious and provide the right amount of vitamins, minerals, and other essential nutrients that our bodies need to stay healthy. Reading food labels can help us make these smart food choices. Food labels provide information about the ingredients in a food product, as well as the serving size and nutritional content. By paying attention to these labels, we can make more informed decisions about what we eat.

For example, if we are trying to limit our intake of sodium, we can use the information on a food label to choose foods that are lower in sodium. Or if we are trying to increase our intake of fiber, we can look for foods that are higher in fiber. Overall, making smart food choices and reading food labels can help us make healthier decisions about our diet and improve our overall well-being.

Here are some tips to help you make better choices and understand the labels on food.

Focus on eating whole, unprocessed, or minimally processed foods as much as you can. These foods have more nutrients and less added ingredients, sugars, and bad fats.

Include different colorful fruits and vegetables in your meals. They have lots of vitamins, minerals, antioxidants, and fiber.

Pick protein sources that have less fat, like chicken, fish, lean meats, beans, tofu, tempeh, and low-fat dairy products. These choices have less unhealthy fats and can help you have a healthy diet.

Choose whole grains such as brown rice, quinoa, oats, and whole wheat instead of refined grains like white rice and white bread. Whole grains have lots of nutrients and fiber that make you healthier.

Be aware of how much food you are eating so that you don't eat too much. Use smaller plates and bowls for your food and pay attention when you feel hungry or full.

When you're looking at labels, make sure to read the list of ingredients. The ingredients are listed from heaviest to lightest, with the most important ingredient listed first. Select items that contain a smaller number of easily recognizable ingredients.

Look at the information on the nutrition label. Pay attention to the serving sizes and the amounts of calories, fats (both saturated and trans fats), sugars, sodium, and fiber.

Watch out for extra sugars: Be careful of sugar that is added to foods and drinks. Select items that have low or no additional sugars and go for naturally sweetened choices whenever you can.

Be careful about how much sodium is in your food. Don't eat too much salt because it can cause problems like high blood pressure and other health issues. Try to find options that have less salt.

Be careful with trans fats: Don't eat foods that have trans fats because they can make your bad cholesterol go up and raise the chances of having heart disease. Make sure to read the list of ingredients and look for "partially hydrogenated oils. "

Look for Allergens: If you are allergic to certain foods or have sensitivities, make sure to read the labels carefully to avoid ingredients that could cause an allergic reaction.

Be careful about food labels that say things like "low-fat," "natural," or "organic. " These claims might not mean that the product is actually healthier.

Always check the nutrition label to find accurate information.

When you choose packaged foods, think about how they fit into your whole diet. Try to have meals that contain a good balance of nutrients like carbohydrates, proteins, and fats, as well as vitamins and minerals.

By paying attention to the food, you choose and look at the labels, you can make smart decisions that help you stay healthy and feel good. It's important to eat a variety of foods and exercise regularly to stay healthy.

Tips for Efficient and Healthy Meal Planning

Planning your meals in a smart and healthy way can help you save time, and money, and reduce stress. It also guarantees that you're providing your body with good and nourishing food.

Here are some suggestions to help you make a good meal plan.

Set aside a specific time each week to plan your meals. This could be during the weekend or any other day that is most convenient for you. Having a set schedule will make it easier to plan meals regularly and handle them easily.

Make a list of what you will eat each day of the week before it starts. Think about the meals we eat in the morning, midday, evening, and also the small foods we have in between. Having a menu will help you plan ahead and make healthier choices by avoiding making sudden decisions.

Use a format or application to plan your meals for the week. This can make the process easier and make sure you eat all types of food every week.

Think about your weekly schedule before planning your meals. If you are busy, pick recipes that are fast and simple to make. When you have extra time, you can make fancier meals.

Eat foods that are packed with nutrients. Try to include a wide range of these nutrient-rich foods in your meals. Include fruits, vegetables, whole grains, lean meats, and healthy fats in your diet for well-rounded and healthy nutrition.

Batch cooking means cooking food in larger quantities at once, especially things like grains, proteins, and sauces. By doing this, you can use the extra food from previous meals for many different meals throughout the week.

Make extra food on purpose so you can eat it the next day for lunch or dinner.

This not only helps you save time but also decreases how much food is wasted.

Make a list of the food you need to buy at the store. When you go shopping, only buy what's on your list so you don't make sudden purchases and can stick to your healthy choices.

Buy in large amounts: Buy items like grains, beans, nuts, and seeds in big quantities to save money and create less waste from packaging.

Get ready ahead of time by washing, cutting, and preparing ingredients like vegetables and fruits. Having all the necessary ingredients ready beforehand will make cooking meals faster and easier.

Be open to changing your meals even if you have a plan. Life is full of surprises and things may not always go as planned. Be willing to change if necessary.

Get your family members to help plan meals if you can. Ask people for their opinions and take into account what they like when preparing meals to ensure that everyone enjoys their food.

Try new recipes and use different ingredients to see what happens. Change up your favorite dishes to make them more interesting.

By using these tips, you can make your meal planning easier and make sure you're eating tasty and healthy meals all week. Make sure to understand that meal planning gets better when you do it more often, so don't rush it and find a routine that suits you and your daily life.

Tips for Eating Healthy Eating

Here are some strategies to help you eat healthier:

Eating healthy is really important for staying in good health and feeling well. Using the right techniques can help you to stay committed to a healthy eating plan.

Prioritize Whole Foods: Choose whole, unprocessed, or minimally processed foods whenever possible. These foods are typically more nutrient-dense and contain fewer additives, sugars, and unhealthy fats.

Incorporate Fruits and Vegetables: Aim to include a variety of colorful fruits and vegetables in your diet. They are rich in vitamins, minerals, antioxidants, and fiber.

Choose Lean Proteins: Chose sources of protein, such as poultry, fish, lean cuts of meat, legumes, tofu, tempeh, and low-fat dairy products. These options are lower in saturated fats and can contribute to a balanced diet.

Include Whole Grains: Select whole grains like brown rice, quinoa, oats, and whole wheat over refined grains (e.g., white rice, white bread). Whole grains retain more nutrients and fiber, promoting better overall health.

Mindful Portion Sizes: Pay attention to portion sizes to avoid overeating. Use smaller plates and bowls, and listen to your body's hunger and fullness cues.

Read Ingredient Lists: When reading labels, check the ingredient list. Ingredients are listed in descending order by weight, with the most prominent ingredient listed first. Choose products with fewer recognizable ingredients.

Check Nutritional Information: Examine the nutritional information on the label, paying attention to serving sizes and the content of calories, fats (saturated and trans fats), sugars, sodium, and fiber.

Look for Added Sugars: Be cautious of added sugars in foods and beverages.

Choose products with little or no added sugars, and opt for naturally sweetened options whenever possible.

Watch for Sodium Content: Limit foods high in sodium, as excessive salt intake can contribute to high blood pressure and other health issues. Look for lower-sodium alternatives.

Be Wary of Trans Fats: Avoid products containing trans fats, as they can raise bad cholesterol levels and increase the risk of heart disease. Check the ingredient list for "partially hydrogenated oils."

Check for Allergens: If you have food allergies or sensitivities, carefully read labels to avoid ingredients that may trigger an allergic reaction.

Understand Food Claims: Be cautious of food marketing claims like "low-fat," "natural," or "organic." Some claims may not necessarily indicate a healthier product. Always refer to the nutrition label for accurate information.

Consider the Whole Meal: When selecting packaged foods, think about how they fit into your overall diet. Aim for balanced meals that include a mix of macronutrients and micronutrients.

By becoming more conscious of food choices and reading labels, you can make informed decisions that support your health and well-being. Remember that a diverse, balanced diet, along with regular physical activity, is essential for overall health.

Tips for Efficient and Healthy Meal Planning

Efficient and healthy meal planning can save you time, money, and stress while ensuring that you're nourishing your body with nutritious foods. Here are some tips to help you create a successful meal-planning routine:

Set Aside Dedicated Time: Allocate a specific time each week to plan your meals. This could be on the weekend or any other day that works best for you. Having a consistent schedule will make meal planning a regular and manageable task.

Create a Weekly Menu: Plan your meals for the entire week in advance. Consider breakfasts, lunches, dinners, and snacks. Having a menu will prevent last-minute decisions and reduce the likelihood of opting for less healthy choices.

Use a Template: Develop a meal planning template or use an app to organize your weekly menu. This can help streamline the process and ensure you cover all food groups throughout the week.

Consider Your Schedule: Take your weekly schedule into account when planning meals. If you have a busy day, choose quick and easy recipes. On days when you have more time, you can prepare more elaborate dishes.

Include Nutrient-Dense Foods: Aim to include a variety of nutrient-dense foods in your meals. Incorporate fruits, vegetables, whole grains, lean proteins, and healthy fats to ensure balanced nutrition.

Batch Cooking: Cook in batches and prepare larger portions, especially for items like grains, proteins, and sauces. This way, you can use leftovers for multiple meals during the week.

Plan for Leftovers: Intentionally cook extra food to have leftovers for the next day's lunch or dinner. This not only saves time but also reduces food waste.

Shop with a List: Create a grocery list based on your meal plan. Stick to the list when shopping to avoid impulsive purchases and stay on track with your healthy choices.

Buy in Bulk: Purchase non-perishable items, such as grains, legumes, nuts, and seeds, in bulk to save money and reduce packaging waste.

Prep Ingredients in Advance: Wash, chop, and prep ingredients ahead of time, such as vegetables and fruits. Having prepared ingredients on hand will make cooking meals quicker and more convenient.

Try One-Pot or Sheet Pan Meals: Look for recipes that require minimal cooking utensils and cleanup. One-pot or sheet pan meals can simplify your cooking process.

Stay Flexible: While it's essential to plan, be flexible with your meals. Life can be unpredictable, and plans may change. Be open to making adjustments if needed.

Involve the Family: If possible, involve your family members in meal planning. Get their input and consider their preferences to make meals enjoyable for everyone.

Experiment and Rotate Recipes: Don't be afraid to try new recipes and experiment with different ingredients. Rotate your favorite meals to keep things exciting.

By following these tips, you can streamline your meal planning process and ensure that you're nourishing your body with delicious and nutritious meals throughout the week. Remember, meal planning is a skill that improves with practice, so be patient and find a routine that works best for you and your lifestyle.

Healthy Eating Strategies

Healthy eating is a fundamental aspect of maintaining good health and well-being. Adopting the right strategies can make it easier to stick to a nutritious diet. Here are some healthy eating strategies:

Tips for Healthy Eating

Eating healthy is very important for our health and overall well-being. Using the correct strategies can make it simpler to stick to a healthy diet. Here are some tips to eat healthily:

Try to eat a balanced diet with different types of foods from all food groups, like fruits, vegetables, whole grains, lean proteins, and healthy fats. To avoid eating too much, try to have moderate amounts of food.

Eat more foods that are high in fiber like fruits, veggies, whole grains, and legumes. Fiber is good for your digestion and makes you feel less hungry for a longer time.

Be careful with how much salt you eat: Eat less salt by not eating foods that have a lot of salt added, like processed foods. Use herbs and spices to add flavor to your food instead of using salt. Limit intake of processed and sugary foods.

Choose whole foods, such as fruits, vegetables, whole grains, lean meats, and low-fat dairy products.

Control portion sizes to avoid overeating. Watch how much you eat. Be aware of how big your portions are. To stop eating too much, use smaller plates and don't eat straight from big packages.

Drink plenty of water and limit sugary beverages. To stay hydrated, make sure to drink lots of water during the day. Don't drink too many sugary drinks, choose water or drinks without added sugar instead.

Plan and prepare meals in advance to avoid unhealthy food choices.

Listen to your body's hunger and fullness cues.

Incorporate regular physical activity to maintain a healthy lifestyle.

Remember, making small, sustainable changes in your eating habits can lead to long-term health benefits.

Everyone has different nutritional needs, so it's important to find a healthy eating plan that works well for you and can be continued for a long time. If you have particular health worries or dietary limitations, it might be helpful to talk to a registered dietitian or healthcare professional for individualized advice.

Chapter 4

Mindful Eating

Mindful eating means being fully present and aware while eating. It means paying close attention to how the food looks, smells, tastes, and makes us feel. It also involves being aware of our thoughts and emotions while eating. It means being aware of the present moment without judging it. This practice encourages people to eat intentionally and be aware of their eating habits. It can help improve their relationship with food and make eating a more meaningful experience.

Eating mindfully means focusing on your meal without being distracted by things like phones and TVs. It involves chewing your food slowly and well, and really noticing the tastes and textures of what you're eating. It's important to eat when you are hungry and stop when you are full, instead of eating because you are used to or bored.

Remember, when we talk about mindful eating, we are not talking about following strict diets or limiting the food we can eat. Instead, it is about developing a good and aware connection with food, which helps us adopt a healthier way of eating and overall happiness.

Understanding the Mind-Body Connection in Eating

The mind-body connection when it comes to eating means that our thoughts, emotions, and actions related to food can affect our physical health. This connection emphasizes how our thoughts and emotions affect the way we eat, digest food, and our overall well-being. By recognizing and taking advantage of this connection, we can have a better and healthier approach to eating.

Here are a few important things to know about how your mind and body are connected when it comes to eating:

Emotional eating: Our feelings greatly affect how and what we eat. Feeling stressed, sad, bored, or other strong emotions can lead to emotional eating. This means people may eat food to seek comfort or distraction, even if they aren't actually hungry.

Mindful eating means paying close attention to what we eat and how it makes us feel. It helps us connect our mind and body. By paying attention and being mindful during meals, we can better notice when we're hungry, when we're full, and when our emotions make us want to eat.

Stress and Digestion: When you're really stressed out, it can make your digestion not work as well. When we feel stressed, our body reacts by activating the "fight or flight" response. This causes less energy to be used for digestion. This can cause problems with digestion like feeling full or uncomfortable in the stomach.

Gut-Brain Axis: The gut-brain axis is a two-way communication system between the gut and the brain. The stomach has a complicated system of nerves and chemicals that some people call the "second brain". This connection between the stomach and brain affects our feelings, emotions, and even the choices we make, which can then impact how we eat.

Body Image and Eating Disorders: Body image problems can cause people to develop unhealthy eating habits. Feeling bad about how your body looks and not feeling good about yourself can make you eat very little, eat a lot at once, or develop other problems with eating.

Cultural and Social Influences: Our cultural background and the people around us can greatly affect the type of food we decide to eat and how we eat it. The way we think about and eat food can be influenced by what is considered normal in society, our family's customs, and the opinions of our friends.

Nutrition and Mental Health: Eating good food is important for our mental health. Consuming diets that contain lots of fruits, vegetables, whole grains, and healthy fats has been linked to improved mood and thinking abilities.

Psychological Health and Weight Management

Mental health can affect how well we manage our weight. Feeling stressed, sad, or worried can mess with your hormones, like cortisol, which might make you gain weight or make it harder for you to lose weight.

Understanding how our thoughts and feelings are connected to our eating habits can give us the ability to make better choices about the food we eat and form healthier eating routines. Here are some ways to help your body and mind connect when eating:

Try to be more aware of when you are hungry or full, and what might make you eat even when you're not hungry.

Discover different ways to handle your feelings without using food as a crutch.

Develop a good opinion of your own body and be kind to yourself.

Learn to relax and reduce stress by doing activities like meditation, taking deep breaths, or practicing yoga.

In simpler terms, knowing how our thoughts and feelings affect our eating habits helps us have a healthy and appreciative attitude towards food that benefits both our bodies and minds.

Practicing Mindful Eating for Greater Satisfaction and Awareness

Learning to eat mindfully can bring you more pleasure and help you become more aware of your eating habits.

Eating mindfully can help you enjoy and pay attention to your meals more. Here are some specific ways to help you practice mindful eating every day:

Eat without any distractions: Make sure you are in a quiet and focused eating area by switching off the TV, keeping your phone away, and not getting distracted by anything else. This helps you focus completely on your meal.

Engage Your Senses: Before you eat, take a second to look at and smell your food. Pay attention to the colors, textures, and smells. Using your senses can make eating more enjoyable.

Chew Slowly and Thoroughly: Take your time and chew your food slowly and carefully. Enjoy every bite and pay attention to the taste. This not only helps your body break down food but also lets you fully experience the tastes and enjoy them.

Put Down Your Utensils: Please rest your utensils between each bite. When you take a short break, it helps you concentrate on the food in your mouth instead of mindlessly eating.

Tune into Hunger and Fullness Cues: Pay attention to your body's signals of hunger and fullness. Take note of when you are genuinely hungry and when you feel satisfied and not overly full. Mindful eating means only eating when you are hungry and stopping when you feel full and satisfied.

Observe Emotional Eating Triggers: Pay attention to the things that make you want to eat because of your emotions. If you eat when you're not hungry, stop and think about how you're feeling. Then, find other ways to deal with those emotions instead of using food.

Practice Mindful Drinking: Try to be mindful of what you drink. No matter what you're drinking, like water, tea, or coffee, try to enjoy the flavor and temperature as you take each sip.

Begin by taking small steps: Start with having one meal a day or even just being mindful of what you eat during snack times. As you get more used to it, you can start doing it for more meals.

Just keep in mind that being mindful about what you eat doesn't mean you have to be perfect or overly strict with your food choices. It's about being aware of how you eat without judging yourself and improving your relationship with food to make it healthier and more enjoyable. Like any other mindfulness activity, it might take time and patience to get used to mindful eating. However, it can have a big positive impact on your physical and mental health.

Overcoming Emotional Eating and Food Cravings

Overcoming emotional eating and cravings for food can be difficult but it is important for having a healthy and balanced relationship with what we eat. Here are some ways to help you control eating when you're emotional and lessen your desire for food.

Find out what causes emotional eating or food cravings by paying attention to your emotions, situations, or things that stress you out. Writing down what you eat in a journal can help you see how you eat and understand your eating habits better.

Instead of using food to make yourself feel better or take your mind off things, you should try finding different ways to deal with your feelings. Take part in things that make you happy, like working out, sitting quietly, writing in a journal, being with people you care about, or doing things you enjoy.

Try to be present and aware while eating, as it can help you overcome eating based on emotions. Before you eat, stop for a moment and think about whether you are really hungry or if there are other reasons, like emotions, that are making you want to eat. Eat your food slowly, enjoy each bite, and be aware of when you are hungry and when you are full.

Create a helpful atmosphere by being around friends, family, or a support group that can assist you during tough times and motivate your healthy eating choices.

If there are foods that always make you eat when you feel emotional or have strong cravings, you should try to have less of those foods around you at home or at work. Instead, make sure you have healthier options easily accessible.

Managing stress is important because it often leads to emotional eating and cravings. Try doing activities like yoga, deep breathing, or meditation to help you feel less stressed.

Make sure to get enough sleep. Not getting enough sleep can make you feel hungrier and have strong desires for food. Make sure you are getting enough good sleep every night to help maintain healthy eating habits.

Eat a mix of different healthy foods like fruits, vegetables, whole grains, lean meats, and good fats to have a balanced diet. Eating a well-balanced diet can help keep your blood sugar steady and decrease your desire for unhealthy snacks.

Sometimes, not having enough water in your body can make you think you are hungry or have a strong desire for food. Make sure to drink plenty of water during the day to stay hydrated.

If you can't control your emotional eating or food cravings by yourself and it's a constant problem, you should think about getting help from a registered dietitian, therapist, or counselor who knows about eating disorders and emotional eating.

Take your time and be nice to yourself while going through this process. Celebrate when you do something good, even if it's small, and continue working towards having a better and more balanced relationship with food.

Chapter 5

Cooking for Health and Flavor

Learning and becoming skilled at basic cooking methods can greatly improve your ability to make nutritious and tasty meals. Here are some basic cooking techniques to focus on:

Sauteing means cooking food fast in a bit of oil or butter on high heat. It's a flexible method used for cooking vegetables, meat, or seafood.

Steaming is a way of cooking that is gentle and keeps the nutrients in vegetables, fish, and other delicate foods. You can use a special basket for steaming or make your own steamer using a pot and a lid that fits well.

Grilling is a healthy cooking method where you cook food like meat, fish, and vegetables. It helps get rid of extra fat by allowing it to drip away. To cook, you can use a grill pan or an outdoor grill. Make sure to avoid cooking your food until it becomes black or burnt.

Baking and roasting are good ways to cook meat and vegetables in the oven. It doesn't need much fat added, so it's healthier.

Boiling is a simple way to cook pasta, grains, and some vegetables. Be cautious not to cook vegetables for too long, because it can cause them to lose their nutrients.

Blanching is a cooking method where you quickly boil vegetables and then put them into cold water to stop them from cooking further. This technique keeps the bright color and freshness of vegetables.

Stir-frying is a fast and effective way to cook small food pieces on high heat. Use a little bit of oil and keep the ingredients moving so they don't get stuck.

Poaching is when you cook food by simmering it in liquid, like water or broth. This is a good way to cook eggs, fish, or chicken breasts in a healthy way.

Marinating is the process of soaking food in tasty liquid before cooking it. It not only makes food taste better but also makes the meat more tender and adds moisture.

Learning how to use herbs, spices, and condiments can make your food taste better without using too much salt or unhealthy fats.

Tips for Healthy Cooking

Use cooking oils like olive oil, avocado oil, or coconut oil, but don't use too much.

Choose healthier protein options like chicken, turkey, fish, and beans.

Make sure to eat different kinds of colorful fruits and vegetables with your meals to get a lot of different nutrients.

Try not to use processed ingredients and choose fresh, whole foods whenever you can.

Try using different herbs and spices to make your food taste better without using too much salt.

To prevent eating too much, make sure to watch and limit the amount of food you eat at a time.

Don't forget, cooking gets better when you keep practicing. Begin with easy recipes and slowly push yourself to attempt new skills and meals. When you cook at home, you get to choose what ingredients to use and how to cook them, which helps you make healthy and well-rounded meals that taste good and fit your diet.

Using herbs and spices in cooking

Adding herbs and spices to your cooking can make your food taste better and also give you lots of health benefits. Here are some easy tips for using herbs and spices effectively in your cooking:

Use fresh herbs instead of dried ones as much as you can. Fresh herbs taste better and smell stronger. If possible, think about growing your own herbs at home.

Match herbs and spices with certain ingredients for the best flavor. For instance, basil tastes good when paired with tomatoes, cilantro is a good match for Mexican food, and rosemary adds great flavor to roasted meats. Try different mixes to see what you like the best.

You can use dried herbs when you are cooking something for a long time. Dried herbs will give more flavor to your dish because they have more time to mix in. Put them in the meal at the beginning of cooking.

Put fresh herbs in your dish just before you finish cooking it. Fresh herbs have delicate tastes that can be made weaker if cooked for too long. Put them in at the end of cooking or sprinkle them on top right before serving.

Toasting whole spices before grinding or using them can make their flavors stronger. Take a skillet and heat it without any oil. Put the spices in the skillet and cook them for a minute or two until they start to smell good.

Control the amounts of herbs and spices you add to your food. Begin with small quantities and try the food as you add more ingredients to make sure the flavors are well-balanced.

Think about how herbs and spices can be good for your health. They have special properties that can help fight against harmful things in your body and decrease inflammation. Turmeric contains a compound called curcumin, which helps reduce inflammation.

Keep dried herbs and spices in sealed containers in a cool, dark place. Make sure to regularly check the expiration dates of whatever you're talking about, because they become less powerful as time goes on.

Try using spices instead of a lot of salt to make your food taste better. This will help you make your food healthier without losing its delicious flavor.

You can try using infused oils and vinegar to add flavors of herbs and spices to your food. You can use them to make dressings, and marinades, or pour them on top of already prepared dishes.

Keep in mind that everyone has different taste preferences, so you can change the amounts and combinations of herbs and spices to match what you like. By practicing and trying different things, you will gain more confidence in using herbs and spices to make tasty and nutritious meals.

Tasty and healthy recipes for all meals.

Adding herbs and spices to your cooking can make your food taste better and also be good for your health. Here are some suggestions on how to use herbs and spices well in your cooking:

Use fresh herbs instead of dried ones whenever you can. Fresh herbs taste and smell stronger. If possible, think about planting and growing your own herbs in your own house.

Use herbs and spices that go well with certain ingredients. For instance, basil tastes good with tomatoes, cilantro tastes good with Mexican food, and rosemary tastes good with roasted meats. Try different combinations to see what you like the most.

You should use dried herbs when you are cooking something for a long time because the flavors from the herbs will have more time to blend into the dish. Put them in the cooking early.

To keep the delicate flavors of fresh herbs strong, it is best to add them to your dish toward the end of the cooking process. Put them in towards the end of cooking or on top just before you serve the food.

Toast whole spices by heating them before grinding or using them. This can make their flavors stronger. Use a pan without oil on medium heat and stir the spices for a minute or two until they start to smell nice.

Be aware of how much herbs and spices you use to balance the flavors. Begin with a small quantity and try it bit by bit to get a good balance of flavors.

Try different ready-made spice mixes from different types of food or make your own special spice mixes. This can make your dishes more interesting and flavorful.

Think about the good things these herbs and spices can do for your health. They have antioxidants, anti-inflammatory properties, and other qualities that can benefit your body. For instance, turmeric contains curcumin, which is known for reducing inflammation.

Chapter 6

Eating Smart on the Go

Eating healthy while busy can be hard. However, if you plan ahead and prepare, you can still make good food choices. Here are some suggestions to eat healthily when you are busy:

Get ready and bring with your healthy snacks that are full of good nutrients. Examples of these snacks are sliced fruits, vegetables, nuts, or granola bars. Having these things available will stop you from choosing unhealthy foods when you're hungry.

When you eat out or get food to go, choose dishes made with whole foods. These can include salads, grilled meats, and sandwiches made with whole-grain bread. Stay away from foods that have been heavily processed and cooked in a lot of oil.

Drink enough water throughout the day by carrying a water bottle that you can use again and again. Don't drink sugary drinks, choose water, herbal teas, or unsweetened drinks instead.

Look up the menu of a restaurant before you go there to eat. Search for locations that have healthier options on their menu or give you the freedom to make your meal the way you like it.

Remember to control how much you eat when you are dining out or getting food to go. Think about sharing big meals with a friend or saving half for another time.

Make sure you always have a set of reusable cutleries (fork, knife, and spoon) with you, either in your bag or car. This way, you won't need to use disposable plastic utensils when you eat while traveling or on the move.

Prepare meals ahead of time: Set aside a little time each week to plan and pack your lunches or dinners in containers. This will make it simpler to quickly grab a healthy meal when you're busy.

When choosing a vending machine, it's better to pick healthier snacks like nuts, whole-grain crackers, or dried fruits instead of sugary snacks and sodas.

Skipping breakfast is not a good idea. Eating a healthy breakfast in the morning can help you make better food choices for the rest of the day. You could try making overnight oats or putting together smoothie packs for fast and easy breakfasts.

Bring small containers of healthier condiments like hummus, salsa, or

Greek yogurt dressing to enhance the taste of your meals without adding too many calories and unhealthy fats.

Make healthy snacks by choosing foods that have protein, fiber, and healthy fats. For instance, you can eat apple slices with peanut butter or carrot sticks with hummus.

Pay attention to when you feel hungry or full. Don't eat without thinking and only eat when you're hungry. Stop eating when you feel full.

Don't forget, eating healthy when you're busy is all about making wise decisions and thinking ahead. You can keep your body healthy and provide it with good nutrition by following these tips every day, even when you're busy.

Making healthy choices when you are eating out or traveling

It can be hard to pick healthy options when eating out or traveling, but with careful planning and decision-making, it is definitely doable. Here are some tips to help you stick to your health goals when eating out or traveling:

Before you go on a trip or plan to eat out, make sure to search for restaurants or places to eat that have healthier choices on their menu. Lots of restaurants have menus online so you can see if they have healthier food options before you go there.

Choose meals that have a mix of different vegetables and fruits. These foods that are packed with nutrients are important for a meal that has a good balance.

Eat foods that are cooked by grilling, steaming, or broiling instead of frying. This makes your meal have fewer bad fats and fewer calories.

Some salads and dishes can have a lot of calories because of high-calorie dressings and sauces. Ask for dressings and sauces separately or ask for healthier options.

Select lean sources of protein such as grilled chicken, fish, or tofu. These choices give your body the important nutrients it needs, without giving it too much of the bad fats that can be harmful.

Avoid drinking sugary drinks like soda or sweetened fruit juices. Instead, go for water, unsweetened tea, or sparkling water.

Be careful when choosing appetizers and desserts because they can make your meal have more calories and unhealthy ingredients. If you want to enjoy something, think about sharing it with others so that you don't eat too much.

Bring healthy snacks when you are traveling. Snacks like nuts, granola bars, or dried fruits are good choices. This will help you avoid unhealthy snacks during long journeys.

Begin your day with a healthy breakfast, even when you're away from home. Lots of hotels have healthier choices for breakfast like oatmeal, yogurt, and fresh fruits.

Stay away from fast food because it is usually not good for your health and doesn't offer healthy options. Find other places like salad bars or markets that offer healthier options that you can take away.

It's fine to have a nice meal or try out local food when you're traveling or eating out. Just try to limit yourself and make healthier choices throughout the day.

When eating out or traveling, it's important to think about what you're choosing to eat and make sure you eat a good mix of different foods. Plan ahead and make smart choices so you can still take care of your body when you're not at home.

Chapter 7

Hydration and Wellness

Drinking enough water is very important for staying healthy and feeling good. Our bodies are mostly made of water, about 60%. It is very important for our bodies to have enough water for everything to work properly.

Keep in mind that how much water your body needs can change depending on different things like your body, how much you move around, and the surroundings you are in. Pay attention to when your body feels thirsty and try your best to drink enough water to stay healthy and feel good.

Why It's Important to Drink Enough Water for Your Health and How It Impacts Your Performance

It is extremely important to drink enough water for good health and to do well at activities or tasks. Water is very important for our body to work properly. Not having enough water, even just a little, can really affect how our body functions. Here are some important reasons why it is essential to stay hydrated for good health and performance:

Water assists in maintaining body temperature by releasing heat through sweating. It is very important to drink enough water to stay hydrated during exercise or when you are in a hot place so that you do not get too hot and avoid getting sick from the heat.

Being properly hydrated means having enough blood in your body. This helps to efficiently carry oxygen and nutrients to your cells and tissues. This is really important for keeping up energy levels and helping with the body's overall functions.

Electrolytes like sodium, potassium, calcium, and magnesium are important for keeping our cells working properly. Drinking enough water is important for keeping your body's electrolytes balanced. When your electrolytes are balanced, your nerves work properly, your muscles can contract, and your fluids stay at the right levels.

Dehydration can make it harder to perform well and have enough energy during exercise. This can make you feel like you are working harder, have less energy to exercise, and are more likely to feel tired and get muscle cramps.

When you are dehydrated, it can harm how your brain works, such as how well you remember things, pay attention and focus. Drinking enough water helps your brain work better and keeps you focused.

Water helps to keep our joints moving smoothly and protects our muscles and organs by providing a cushion. It is important to drink enough water to keep your joints mobile and lower the chance of getting hurt during exercise.

Water helps in getting rid of waste and toxins from the body, mainly through pee and sweat. Drinking enough water helps your kidneys work properly and helps your body get rid of waste.

Drinking enough water every day can help keep your immune system strong. Water helps the body make and move immune cells, which protect against infections and diseases.

Water helps your body properly break down and absorb nutrients from the food you eat, which is important for good digestive health. It also helps stop problems with going to the bathroom and keeps your stomach and guts healthy.

Taking care of your skin is important for its health. One way to do this is by making sure your skin is properly hydrated. When your skin is hydrated, it reduces the chances of it becoming dry, flaky, or having other skin problems.

To keep your body properly hydrated

Remember to drink water often throughout the day, even if you don't feel thirsty.

Check the color of your urine if it is a light-yellow color, it means you are well-hydrated. But if it is a dark yellow color, it means you are dehydrated.

Drink water before, during, and after you exercise or do physical activities.

Think about drinking or eating things with lots of electrolytes when you're exercising a lot or for a long time.

Drink less coffee, tea, and alcohol because they can make you dehydrated.

Keep in mind that each person needs a different amount of water depending on their size, how active they are, and the weather. Pay attention to when your body tells you it is thirsty and make sure to drink enough water to stay healthy, feel good, and perform at your best.

Beyond Water: Exploring Hydrating Foods and Beverages

Looking for foods and drinks that help keep you hydrated is a good idea, especially in hot weather or when you're doing exercise.

These foods and drinks not only taste good and make you feel refreshed, but they also have important nutrients that help keep you healthy. Here are some ways to stay hydrated:

Foods that help keep your body hydrated

Cucumbers are very hydrating vegetables because they contain about 95% water. They have fewer calories and lots of vitamins and minerals.

Watermelon is a yummy and refreshing fruit that is mostly made up of water, about 92%. Tomato is also packed with vitamins A and C, as well as antioxidants such as lycopene. They have a lot of vitamin C, which helps the immune system.

Strawberries are made up of mostly water and also have lots of important vitamins, fiber, and antioxidants.

Lettuce is a type of vegetable that is often used in salads. It has a lot of water in it, especially types like iceberg and romaine.

Celery is a type of vegetable that has a lot of water in it. It is a crispy snack that helps keep you hydrated.

Bell peppers, specifically the ones that have lots of water like green and red peppers, can hydrate you and give you important vitamins.

Cantaloupe is a delicious fruit that is very hydrating, as it contains around 89% water. It is also a healthy way to get vitamin A and potassium.

Drinks that provide hydration

Water is the healthiest drink to keep your body hydrated. It has no calories and is important for staying healthy and hydrated.

Coconut water is a natural drink with lots of electrolytes, which can help replace fluids and important minerals after working out.

Herbal teas are drinks made from plants that have different tastes. When you drink them without adding sugar, they can help keep you hydrated.

Make your water taste better and fresh by putting pieces of fruits like lemon, lime, or berries, or herbs like mint or basil into it.

Make a drink by mixing sliced cucumbers, lemon juice, water, and a small amount of honey. It will keep you hydrated and feel rejuvenating.

To make a watermelon smoothie, blend pieces of watermelon with ice and a little lime juice for a refreshing and tasty drink that helps keep you hydrated.

Make sure to pick drinks that don't have extra sugar and try not to have too many drinks with caffeine or alcohol, since they can make you dehydrated.

If you eat and drink these hydrating foods every day, it will help keep you hydrated and healthy, especially when it's hot outside or you're being active.

Signs of Dehydration and Ways to Stay Hydrated

Signs of not having enough water in your body can be different depending on how serious it is, but some common signs include:

Thirst is when your body tells you that it needs more fluids. If you are thirsty, it means you might be a little bit dehydrated.

When your urine is a dark yellow or amber color and you don't pee very often, it means you are not drinking enough water and you are dehydrated. When you drink enough water, your pee is light yellow.

When your body does not have enough water, it can cause your mouth and throat to feel dry. This can make it hard and uncomfortable to swallow.

Not drinking enough fluids can make you feel tired and weak.

Feeling dizzy or lightheaded can happen when you are dehydrated and it affects your blood pressure.

A headache can happen when you are not getting enough water and become a little dehydrated.

When your body doesn't have enough water, your skin can feel dry, cool, and not as stretchy.

Sometimes, not having enough water in your body can make your heart beat faster.

To keep your body hydrated and avoid dehydration, remember these helpful tips

Drink water often: Try to drink water consistently throughout the day, even if you're not feeling thirsty.

Take a water bottle that you can use again and again with you, so you can easily get water whenever you need it, no matter where you are.

Drink water before you start feeling thirsty because feeling thirsty means you are already dehydrated. Make sure to drink water regularly, especially when it's hot outside or when you're doing physical activities.

Drink water before, during, and after exercising to replenish fluids lost from sweating.

Add watery fruits and veggies such as watermelon, cucumber, oranges, and lettuce to your meals.

Drink less coffee and alcohol because they can make you become dehydrated.

Use alarms or apps on your phone to remind yourself to drink water regularly, especially if you often forget.

Think about keeping the right amount of minerals in your body when you do a lot of exercise. Drink or eat something with electrolytes to help with this.

Drink enough water when you travel, especially during long flights or journeys.

Remember, the amount of water each person needs may be different depending on their body size, how active they are, and the environment they are in. Pay attention to when your body feels thirsty and make sure to drink enough water to stay healthy and feel good. If you have really bad symptoms of dehydration or you can't drink enough to get hydrated, go see a doctor as soon as possible.

Chapter 8

Fitness and Nutrition Synergy

Exercise and eating well have a connected and beneficial relationship. They work together to improve your overall health, well-being, and how well you perform. When fitness and nutrition are used together, they support and benefit each other. Staying fit and eating healthy are both important for a good and healthy life. The combination of these two things improves both our physical and mental health, helps us feel good overall, and helps us form good habits for a balanced and fulfilling life.

Combining exercise and healthy eating in everyday life can bring about significant and beneficial changes in a person's life.

The Connection Between Nutrition and Physical Activity

Good nutrition and physical activity are very important for your health and feeling good. These two things work together to help with different body functions and make a person healthy, energetic, and have a good life. Here's how what you eat and how much you move are connected:

Energy balance refers to the way nutrition gives our body the energy it needs to do things like exercise and move around. The energy we get from the food we eat helps us to exercise and do things in our daily lives. Whether you maintain, gain, or lose weight depends on the balance between the calories you eat and the calories you burn through physical activity.

Having enough good food, especially protein, is really important for keeping our muscles healthy and fixing them when they get hurt. Protein gives our muscles what they need to grow and repair themselves after exercise. Participating in exercise helps our body to use nutrients better, which makes us absorb them more effectively.

Eating the right food is important to do well and last longer in sports and physical activities. Nutrient-rich foods give our bodies the right vitamins, minerals, and carbohydrates to give us energy during workouts and sports.

Nutrition is important for recovering after exercise. Eating the right foods after exercising helps to replace the energy in our muscles, rehydrate our body, and repair our muscles, which lowers the chances of getting tired and getting hurt.

Having enough calcium, vitamin D, and other important nutrients is really important for keeping your bones healthy. Doing physical activities, especially ones that involve putting weight on your bones like walking and doing exercises with resistance, can help keep your bones strong and dense.

Exercising regularly can speed up metabolism, which helps the body burn calories more effectively. Physical activity, when coupled with a well-rounded diet, can help you maintain a healthy weight and body shape.

Maintaining a healthy heart and blood vessels requires both eating good food and staying active. Eating foods like whole grains, fruits, vegetables, and lean proteins that are good for

your heart, and also exercising regularly can lower your chance of getting heart disease.

Eating well and staying active can lower your chances of getting diseases like type 2 diabetes, some cancers, and health problems caused by being overweight.

Living a long and healthy life can be achieved by eating well and exercising regularly. This can improve how long we live and how well we feel in the future. Eating a well-rounded diet that has lots of nutrients can help keep your brain healthy, improve your thinking skills, and help stabilize your mood. Doing exercise regularly can help make you feel less stressed,

Basically, what you eat and how active you are go together to make a healthy lifestyle. They work well together to help different parts of our body do their jobs, keep us healthy, and lower the chances of getting long-term illnesses. By eating healthy foods and exercising regularly every day, people can live a more balanced and healthier life.

Achieving Fitness Goals with a Smart Eating Plan

Achieving your fitness goals is heavily influenced by eating well, matching your physical activity, and taking care of your body's needs. Here are important rules to help you create a healthy eating plan to reach your fitness goals:

Having specific goals for your health, like getting stronger, having more stamina, losing weight, or gaining muscles, will help you know what to eat and plan your meals accordingly.

Eat a variety of foods that have carbohydrates, proteins, and fats to have a well-balanced diet. Each type of food that provides energy and nutrients plays an important role in helping us stay fit and healthy.

Protein is very important for fixing and building muscles, so it is necessary for achieving fitness goals like getting stronger and building muscle. Add healthy sources of protein like chicken, fish, tofu, beans, and low-fat dairy to your meals.

Eating a well-balanced meal or snack before exercising gives you the energy you need to do your best. Think about eating a mix of foods that have carbohydrates and protein around 1 to 3 hours before you exercise.

It is important to drink enough water for your body to function well and recover properly after physical activity. Make sure to drink water all day, and drink even more when you're exercising or when it's hot outside.

Think about when you eat nutrients to help you reach your fitness goals. For example, eating a meal after exercising that has a lot of protein and carbohydrates helps muscles heal and replaces the body's energy stores.

Be careful about how much you eat so that you don't eat too many calories. Pay attention to how much you eat, especially if you want to lose weight.

Don't avoid healthy fats that come from avocados, nuts, seeds, and olive oil. These fats are important for many body functions and help you feel full.

Stay away from processed foods that contain lots of added sugars, bad fats, and salt. Choose foods that are whole and have a lot of nutrients instead.

Being consistent means doing something again and again, without giving up. It is really important if you want to be successful. Keep following your healthy eating plan for a long time to slowly make progress toward your fitness goals.

Pay attention to how your body reacts to different foods and adjust your eating plan accordingly. Everyone's body may need different types and amounts of food, so what is good for one person might not be good for another.

Keep in mind that achieving your fitness goals involves eating healthy, exercising regularly, and making good choices in your everyday life. It's important to be patient, stay dedicated, and get help from a registered dietitian or nutritionist if you need personal advice and support.

Chapter 9

Special Dietary Consideration

Meeting Nutritional Needs Without Animal Products

Meeting Nutritional Needs Without Animal Products can be done by eating a variety of plant-based foods that contain all the necessary nutrients.

It is possible to meet your nutritional needs without eating animal products by following a well-thought-out and balanced diet that is based on plants. A diet based on plants can give your body everything it needs to stay healthy, like protein, iron, calcium, omega-3 fatty acids, and vitamins like B12. Here are some important tips to make sure you meet all your nutritional needs when following a plant-based diet:

Eat different kinds of plant-based proteins in your meals. Some examples are beans, lentils, chickpeas, tofu, tempeh, edamame, nuts, seeds, quinoa, and amaranth.

Choose plant-based foods that are high in iron, like lentils, beans, tofu, tempeh, quinoa, fortified cereals, and dark leafy greens such as spinach and kale. Eating vitamin C-rich foods like oranges, peppers, or tomatoes along with iron-rich foods can help your body absorb more iron.

Choosing calcium-fortified plant-based milk, like almond or soy milk, and calcium-set tofu will provide you with sources of calcium. Also, make sure to eat foods that have a lot of calcium in them. Some examples include broccoli, kale, collard greens, orange juice with extra calcium added, and plant-based yogurts with extra calcium added.

Include foods like flaxseeds, chia seeds, hemp seeds, walnuts, and algae-based supplements to get omega-3 fatty acids.

Vitamin B12 is mainly present in animal products. So, if you don't consume animal products, you can still get B12 by including fortified plant-based foods like cereals, plant-based milk, and nutritional yeast in your diet. If you need it, ask your doctor about taking B12 supplements.

To make sure you get all the important building blocks for your body, include different sources of protein that work well together in your meals throughout the day. For instance, putting together beans with rice, hummus with whole-grain pita bread, or tofu with quinoa.

Try eating different types of fruits, vegetables, grains, nuts, seeds, and legumes to get lots of different nutrients.

Make sure to have a variety of healthy foods in your meals. Include things like carbohydrates, proteins, good fats, and lots of different fruits and vegetables.

Pay attention to the information on food labels to find out which products have important nutrients like B12, calcium, and vitamin D added to them.

If you have particular worries about what you eat or any health issues, it's a good idea to talk to a registered dietitian. They can create a special eating plan for you based on plants that suit your individual needs.

Don't forget that choosing to eat only plants is a way of living, and it's important to do it with an understanding of what nutrients you need. When you have a well-thought-out plan, eating a diet based on plants can be healthy and good for both your own well-being and the world around you.

Ensuring a Safe Management of Dietary Restrictions

It is very important to handle dietary restrictions carefully in order to make sure you are getting the right nutrients and avoiding any foods that may cause bad reactions or health problems. If you have food allergies, intolerances, religious dietary restrictions, or follow a specific type of diet (like vegetarian or vegan), here are some tips to help you safely manage your dietary restrictions.

Learn about the types of food you should stay away from and the ones that are okay to eat based on your dietary restrictions. Be careful when reading food labels, and learn about hidden ingredients that could cause problems for you.

Make sure to include a variety of nutrients in your meals to keep yourself healthy. Make sure to eat different types of foods from different food groups to get all the different nutrients your body needs.

Cooking at home means making your own meals in your kitchen. When you do this, you have more power over what goes into your food. This can be helpful if you have allergies or need to avoid certain foods, as it reduces the risk of coming into contact with harmful ingredients.

When you go to a restaurant or a party, make sure to clearly tell the people working there or hosting the event if you have any specific foods you can't eat. Kindly inquire about the different food choices and if the dishes may contain any ingredients that can cause allergies.

Identify alternative options for the foods that you should not consume. Sometimes, there are other options that taste and feel the same.

Before you go to a restaurant, check online reviews to see if they can cater to your dietary needs. Find restaurants that other people with similar dietary needs have reviewed positively.

If you're not sure what food will be available at a party or event, bring your own food that you know is safe to eat.

Always carry your allergy medications with you if you have severe food allergies, just in case you accidentally come into contact with something you are allergic to.

If you have food allergies, be careful about mixing food in shared kitchens or restaurants. It's important to stay away from things that can cause allergies.

If you're not sure about getting enough nutrients because of your diet restrictions, talk to a registered dietitian or healthcare professional for help. They can assist in making a safe and healthy meal plan that fits your individual requirements.

When you try new foods or eat at a restaurant, don't automatically think that a specific dish or product is safe. You should always check the ingredients and how the food is prepared.

Dealing with dietary restrictions can be tough, but if you keep trying and have patience, you can find food that is safe and delicious for you.

It is very important for your health and happiness that you handle your dietary restrictions safely. If you make sure to stay informed, plan well, and get help from healthcare professionals when you need it, you can manage your dietary restrictions and have a safe and balanced diet.

Nutrition for Different Life Stages

Nutrition needs vary throughout different life stages as our bodies go through various changes and growth processes. Adequate nutrition during each life stage is crucial for optimal growth, development, and overall health. Here's an overview of nutrition considerations for different life stages:

Infancy (0-12 months)

Breast milk or formula is the primary source of nutrition for infants up to six months old.

Introduce solid foods gradually around six months while continuing breast milk or formula.

Offer a variety of single-ingredient pureed foods to introduce new tastes and textures.

Avoid added sugars, salt, and honey until after the first year.

Toddlerhood (1-3 years)

Encourage self-feeding and offer a variety of foods from all food groups.

Prioritize whole foods over processed snacks.

Limit sugary snacks, fruit juices, and sugary beverages.

Ensure adequate intake of healthy fats for brain development.

Childhood (4-8 years)

Continue to offer a balanced diet with a focus on whole foods, including fruits, vegetables, whole grains, lean proteins, and low-fat dairy.

Encourage regular physical activity to support healthy growth and development.

Limit added sugars, refined carbohydrates, and unhealthy fats.

Adolescence (9-18 years)

Meet the increased energy needs during growth spurts with nutrient-dense foods.

Pay attention to calcium and vitamin D intake for bone health.

Encourage a well-balanced diet to support cognitive function and academic performance.

Avoid skipping meals and prioritize healthy snacks.

Adulthood (19-50 years)

Focus on a varied diet with a balance of macronutrients and micronutrients.

Stay hydrated and limit sugary beverages.

Consider individual nutrient needs, especially during pregnancy and lactation for women.

Older Adulthood (50+ years)

Consume nutrient-dense foods to meet changing nutritional requirements.

Pay attention to calcium and vitamin D intake for bone health.

Ensure sufficient intake of fiber to support digestive health.

Consider vitamin B12 and vitamin D supplements if necessary.

Pregnancy and Lactation

Meet increased calorie and nutrient needs during pregnancy while focusing on nutrient-dense foods.

Ensure sufficient intake of folate, iron, calcium, and omega-3 fatty acids.

Continue taking prenatal vitamins as recommended by healthcare providers.

During lactation, maintain a balanced diet to support milk production and maternal health.

Throughout all life stages, it's essential to maintain a balanced diet that includes a variety of foods from all food groups. Consulting with a registered dietitian or healthcare professional can be beneficial, especially if you have specific dietary concerns or health conditions at any life stage. They can help create personalized nutrition plans that meet your individual needs and support your overall health and well-being.

Chapter 10

Consistency with Healthy Eating

Dealing with Social Pressures and Peer Influence on Eating Habits

It can be difficult to resist social pressures and peer influence when it comes to eating healthy. Here are some tips to help you handle these situations:

Remember to stay focused on your health and nutrition goals. If you want to eat better, stick to a diet, or control your weight, staying focused on your goals can help you say no when your friends pressure you to do something else.

Learn about nutrition and understand why you make certain dietary choices. Understanding why the way you eat is good for you can make you more comfortable explaining your choices to others when necessary.

Believe in yourself when making decisions about what you eat. Trust your gut feelings and have faith in the choices you make for your diet. Keep in mind that each person has different nutritional needs. What might be good for someone else might not be good for you.

Share your food likes and dislikes with your friends or classmates if you feel okay with it. Tell them that you appreciate being with them, but you have certain food preferences that you want to follow.

Show others how your healthy eating habits make you feel better. Your friends might get interested and motivated to make healthier choices as well.

If you're going out to eat with friends, suggest a restaurant that serves food you like to eat or take turns choosing where to eat. By doing this, you can have more power in deciding what food you want to eat.

If you are going to a party where the food might not be what you like to eat, think about bringing your own dish to share with everyone.

Highlight the social part of get-togethers instead of just the food. Have meaningful talks and have fun with your friends without making food the main focus.

If you feel forced to eat something that doesn't go along with your food choices, just say no politely or give a simple explanation without feeling like you have to explain yourself.

Find friends or groups who are supportive and understanding of your eating choices. Having people around you who support your eating habits can make it easier to keep following them.

Create ways to handle peer pressure when it happens. You can try calming yourself down by taking big breaths, imagining yourself doing well, or stepping away from the situation for a while.

It's okay to treat yourself every now and then or change your eating habits when needed. Don't be too tough on yourself if you occasionally stray from your plan.

To handle the effects of what others, think and the influence of friends on how we eat, it's important to be confident, know ourselves well, and be able to stand up for our own choices. By sticking to what you want to achieve, talking openly, and being careful about the decisions you make, you can handle social situations while still focusing on your health and happiness.

Making Healthy Eating a Way of Life

Changing your eating habits to be healthy is a slow and lasting process. It means making choices about what and how much you eat while being mindful of your body's needs. Here are some important rules to follow for a healthy eating lifestyle:

Start by setting goals for your eating habits that are possible to achieve and are practical. Do not follow difficult diets or strict rules, because they are hard to keep up with over a long period of time.

Pay attention to eating whole foods: Choose foods that have not been processed much for your diet. These include fruits, vegetables, grains, lean meats, nuts, seeds, and beans.

To avoid eating too much, make sure to watch how much food you put on your plate. Understand how to pay attention when you feel hungry or full.

Limit the amount of added sugars and salt you consume. Try not to have too much sugar or sodium in your diet. Be careful of the sugars that are not easy to see in packaged foods and choose fruits instead for a natural way to add sweetness.

Remember to drink lots of water throughout the day to stay hydrated. Drink less sugary drinks and try drinking water, herbal teas, or infused water instead.

Make a meal plan ahead of time so that you have healthy food choices ready to eat. This can assist you in resisting the desire to eat unhealthy foods when you are feeling hungry.

Make your own food at home as often as you can. When you cook at home, you can decide what ingredients to use and pick cooking methods that are better for your health.

Pay attention to how you eat, like when you eat because of your emotions or when you snack without thinking. We can encourage better choices by addressing these habits.

Try to eat different types of food so that you get many different nutrients. Try different recipes and types of food to make meals more exciting.

Try to have a good balance in your eating habits, rather than constantly trying to be perfect. It's okay to sometimes treat yourself and enjoy food as long as it is done in a balanced way.

Pay attention to your body: Understand when you feel hungry or full. Eat when you feel hungry, and stop eating when you feel satisfied.

It takes time and energy to change the way you eat. Be kind to yourself and don't judge yourself too harshly. Enjoy and be proud of the improvements you have made. Concentrate on the good things that have happened.

Make sure to keep up-to-date on facts about healthy eating and any recommendations for staying healthy. Knowing a lot about food can help you make smarter decisions about what you eat.

Don't go on super strict diets or eat in very limited ways. Instead, concentrate on creating a long-lasting and pleasant way of eating.

By following these principles every day, you can create a habit of healthy eating. Always remember that adopting a habit of eating healthy is all about taking care of your body, feeling great, and finding happiness in the food you choose to eat.

Chapter 11

Taking Your Health to the Next Level

Here are some important steps to help you improve your health:

Set clear and specific health goals. Make sure they are measurable, achievable, relevant, and have a set timeframe (SMART goals). Having clear goals helps to know what you want to achieve and stay motivated. It could be about getting healthier, losing weight, dealing with stress, or taking care of certain health issues.

It's important to exercise regularly for your overall health. Try to do a combination of exercises that get your heart rate up, exercises that make your muscles stronger, exercises that help you become more flexible, and exercises that help you improve your balance. Discover things that you like to do, because it will be easier to keep doing them regularly.

Eat a variety of healthy foods like fruits, vegetables, whole grains, lean meats, and good fats to have a balanced diet. Reduce the amount of processed foods, sugary drinks, and foods that are high in sodium and unhealthy fats.

Try to be aware of how you eat and be fully engaged in your meals. Paying attention while eating can help you to understand when you are hungry or full, and make better decisions about what to eat.

Continuous stress can harm your health. Include activities that help to reduce stress, like meditation, yoga, deep breathing exercises, or spending time outdoors.

Make sleep a priority and try to have a regular sleep routine. Try to get 7-9 hours of good sleep every night to keep your body and mind healthy.

Make sure to drink lots of water during the day to stay hydrated and help your body work properly.

Stay away from bad habits that can hurt your health. Try to cut down or stop doing things like smoking, drinking too much alcohol, or spending too much time in front of screens.

Regular health checkups are important appointments that you should make with your healthcare provider. During these checkups, your healthcare provider will check on your health, listen to any worries you may have, and give you advice to prevent health problems.

Make sure to spend time with your loved ones and friends for strong relationships. Having people in your life who support and care about you is very important for your mental and emotional health.

Keep up-to-date on information about your health, new studies, and current health patterns. Being knowledgeable about health can give you the ability to make smarter choices for your well-being.

If you have specific health goals or concerns, it's a good idea to ask for help from professionals like dietitians, personal trainers, or mental health therapists.

Please stay calm and keep trying: Getting healthier takes time and effort, so it's important to be patient and keep pushing forward. Take time to appreciate any progress you make, even if it's small. Be gentle with yourself when things don't go as planned.

Keep educating yourself about how to stay healthy, eat well, and stay fit. Knowing things helps you make smart decisions for your health and happiness.

Pay attention to your overall health: Keep in mind that being healthy means more than just not being sick. It means taking care of your body and mind and feeling good in every way. Try to have a balance in everything you do in your life.

Improving your health is a personal and empowering process. If you work hard and take care of yourself, you can improve your health and have a better life.

Exploring Supplements and Their Role in a Balanced Diet

The use of supplements can help support a healthy diet by providing important nutrients that might be missing from the diet or meeting specific health requirements. But remember, supplements are meant to go along with a healthy diet, not take its place. Let's take a closer look at how supplements can be helpful in a healthy diet.

Getting all the necessary nutrients from food alone can be tough for some people. Supplements can help make sure you get all the vitamins, minerals, and other important things your body needs.

Certain people may need to eat more of certain nutrients because of their age, health conditions, or the way they live their lives. For instance, pregnant women may need to take folic acid pills, vegans may need to take vitamin B12 pills, and people who don't get much sun may benefit from taking vitamin D pills.

Supplements are convenient and easy to reach, especially for people who are busy or have limited access to healthy foods.

Certain supplements are created to help with specific health objectives. For example, there are supplements that contain omega-3 fatty acids to improve heart health or probiotics to promote gut health.

People who do intense physical activities can use certain supplements to help improve their performance, recover their muscles, and have more energy overall.

Supplements can help avoid or handle the lack of nutrients, particularly in situations where just changing your diet is not enough.

As people get older, their bodies may require different types of nutrients. Some pills, like calcium and vitamin D, are good for old people's bones.

Some health problems can make it harder for your body to absorb nutrients or cause you to lose nutrients more quickly. In some situations, doctors may give you supplements if you lack certain nutrients.

While supplements can help, it's important to use them wisely and seek advice from a healthcare professional, particularly for high-dose or specialty supplements. Here are some important things to think about:

Some people may require supplements while others may not. Talk to a qualified dietitian or healthcare professional to find out if you need supplements and to figure out which ones are best for you.

Choose well-known brands and check for certifications from independent organizations to make sure the supplements are safe and of good quality.

Do not take too much of supplements. It can cause imbalances and bad effects.

Before relying on supplements, try to get nutrients from whole foods whenever you can. Whole foods have a combination of nutrients and helpful compounds that supplements may not have.

Keep track of your nutrition and check if you need to change the amount of supplements you take based on any changes in your eating habits, daily routine, or overall health.

In summary, supplements can be a helpful addition to a balanced diet when used wisely and according to personal needs. But they should never take the place of a healthy diet that includes many different types of whole, unprocessed foods. Always speak to a knowledgeable healthcare expert before taking any supplements to make sure they are safe and right for your specific health goals and conditions.

Combining Different Approaches to Healthy Eating and Overall Well-being

Using holistic approaches to nutrition and wellness means thinking about how different parts of our health and well-being are connected to make sure our bodies and minds are in balance and working well together. Here are some important ideas and actions that can be used:

Practice being mindful of what you eat by paying attention to the foods you choose, eating at a slow pace, and enjoying every bite. Being mindful and attentive while eating can improve your connection with food and support you in making healthier and more intentional choices.

Eat whole, healthy foods like fruits, vegetables, whole grains, lean meats, nuts, and seeds for good nutrition. These foods have lots of good things in them that help keep you healthy.

Each person has different needs for nutrition. When creating a nutrition plan, think about things like how old you are, if you are a boy or a girl, how much exercise you do, any health problems you have, and what kinds of foods you like.

Encourage a lifestyle where you exercise, get enough rest, manage stress, and make time to relax and take care of yourself.

Try out holistic therapies such as acupuncture, chiropractic care, aromatherapy, or massage to help your body and mind feel better.

Understand how the mind and body are connected and how this connection affects our health. Take part in activities like yoga, meditation, or tai chi to help improve your mental clarity and emotional well-being.

Think about how the food you choose affects the environment. Choose sustainable and environment-friendly practices by opting for locally sourced and organic foods whenever you can.

Be aware of emotional eating and try to find other ways to deal with emotions instead of using food.

Understand how important having a healthy digestive system is for your overall health and well-being. Add foods that are rich in probiotics and fiber to help maintain a healthy community of microorganisms in your gut.

Build positive relationships with others and create a feeling of belonging to a group. Building strong and meaningful connections with others can have a good impact on your mental and emotional well-being.

Herbal remedies are natural medications and supplements that can be used for specific health issues. It's important to consult with trained professionals when using these remedies.

Develop a habit of being thankful for things in life to help you see the good and feel more positive about your well-being.

Get help from professionals who specialize in diet, medicine, or wellness. They can help you incorporate holistic methods into your daily life.

Keep in mind that when talking about nutrition and wellness, holistic approaches focus on the entire person including the body, mind, and spirit. The goal is to find a state of balance and harmony. By following these principles and practices, you can create a well-rounded approach to healthy eating and well-being that helps improve your overall health and happiness.

Chapter 12

How to Stay Healthy for Life

Keep in mind that your path to staying healthy for the rest of your life is special and individual to you. This is about making little but long-lasting changes in order to create a happy and healthy life. Be happy about every little thing you do to become healthier and know that all your hard work is important.

Creating a Sustainable Healthy Lifestyle

Developing a sustainable and healthy lifestyle is an ongoing process that needs dedication and staying consistent. By following these steps every day and making them a regular part of your life, you can slowly develop better habits that will improve your overall health and happiness. It's important to give yourself time and not expect big changes all at once. Small improvements can make a big difference over time. Celebrate your achievements and stay motivated to keep going towards a happier and healthier life. Always remember that every good decision you make is a small but important step towards living a healthy and sustainable life. Here are some important things to do to create a long-lasting and healthy way of living:

Set goals that make sense and are possible to achieve when it comes to your health. Take apart your big goals into smaller, easier steps to prevent getting stressed or overwhelmed.

Pay attention to eating whole, nutrient-rich foods as a priority in your diet. Try to eat a variety of fruits, vegetables, whole grains, lean meats, and good fats in your diet.

Try to be aware of how you eat by listening to your hunger and fullness signals, enjoying your meals, and avoiding anything that might distract you while you're eating.

Make sure to do physical activities regularly in your daily routine. Discover activities that you like to do in order to make exercising a long-lasting and enjoyable routine in your life.

Set up a plan for each day or week that includes time for eating well, staying active, and taking care of yourself.

Being consistent is very important in developing habits that will stay with you for a long time.

Make sure you get a good amount of sleep every night. Create a nighttime routine that helps you relax and sleep better. Discover stress-relieving methods that work well for you, like meditation, taking deep breaths, or spending time outdoors.

Reduce or stop doing things that are bad for you, like smoking, drinking too much alcohol, and spending too much time in front of screens. Stay hydrated by drinking lots of water during the day. This helps keep your body functioning properly.

It is important to be kind to yourself and understand that perfection is not the ultimate aim. Welcome and accept progress, even if it happens slowly, and concentrate on always getting better. Take time to acknowledge and enjoy your achievements, even if they may seem insignificant. Give yourself credit and a treat for sticking to your healthy habits

Learn about health, nutrition, and fitness by reading reliable information and keeping up with the latest research and advice. Be ready to change your healthy lifestyle when necessary. Life is always changing, and sometimes you may need to make changes to your health routine.

Focus on taking care of yourself and doing things that make you happy, help you relax, and make you feel satisfied.

Keep in mind that a long-lasting and healthy lifestyle requires more than just temporary fixes or short-term adjustments. It's about forming habits that you can keep doing for a long time. Take your time, keep working towards your goals, and have fun on your journey to becoming a better and happier version of yourself.

Conclusion

In summary, eating smart and living strong is a transformative journey that puts us on the path to healthier, more fulfilling lives. In this book, we delved deep into the complex relationship between nutrition and overall well-being, discovering the power of conscious food choices to nourish our bodies and minds.

As we read through the pages, we learned that eating smart is more than just following strict diets and counting calories. It is about gaining a deeper understanding of our body's needs and creating a harmonious relationship with the food we consume. By eating a balanced and varied diet high in whole foods, we have seen increased energy levels, stronger immunity, and improved mood.

The book emphasizes the importance of mindful eating and encourages you to savor every bite, savor the taste, and appreciate the way you eat. Practicing this habit helped us better respond to hunger and satiety signals, resulting in a natural and sustainable approach to weight management.

Additionally, Eat Smart and Live Strong emphasizes the long-term health benefits of a lifestyle that emphasizes physical activity and regular exercise. We have seen that incorporating exercise into our daily lives has a huge impact not only on increasing physical fitness but also on mental clarity and emotional well-being.

One of the most important takeaways from this book is that the path to optimal health is not a lonely one. The support of family, friends, and community is essential to the pursuit of lasting change. By creating an environment of encouragement and inspiration, we empower ourselves and those around us to adopt healthier habits together.

Turn to the last page to apply the wisdom of eating smart and living strong to your daily life. Let it guide you in making conscious choices to nourish your body with healthy foods, actively nourish your mind, and participate in activities that energize your mind.

Remember, the path to a healthier, stronger life is about progress, not perfection. It's about embracing small victories, learning from setbacks, and knowing that every step you take brings you one step closer to vitality and a fulfilling life. May 'Eat Smart and Live Strong' become a treasured companion, motivating us to embark on lifelong health adventures, and influence its teachings to create a healthier, happier world for generations to come. Together, let's eat smart, live strong, and thrive in the brilliance of a fulfilling life.